Homemade Lip Balm:

Fun And Unique DIY lipstick And Lip Balm Recipes

Mandy Phan

The Recipes

Coconut Mango Butter Lipstick
Natural Honey Lipstick
Murumuru Butter Lipstick (restores skin elasticity)
Cocoa Butter And Aloe Lip Gloss
DIY Matte Liquid Lip Gloss
Homemade Dreamy Creamy Lip Gloss
Rich Avocado Lip Gloss
DIY Fun Bubble Gum Lipstick
Yummy Sugar Lipstick
DIY Gummy Candy Lipstick
Lipstick Made From Real Fruits And Vegetables
Black Daredevil Lipstick
Natural Peppermint Lip Plumper
DIY EOS Skittles Lip Balm
Holiday Special Candy Cane Lip Gloss

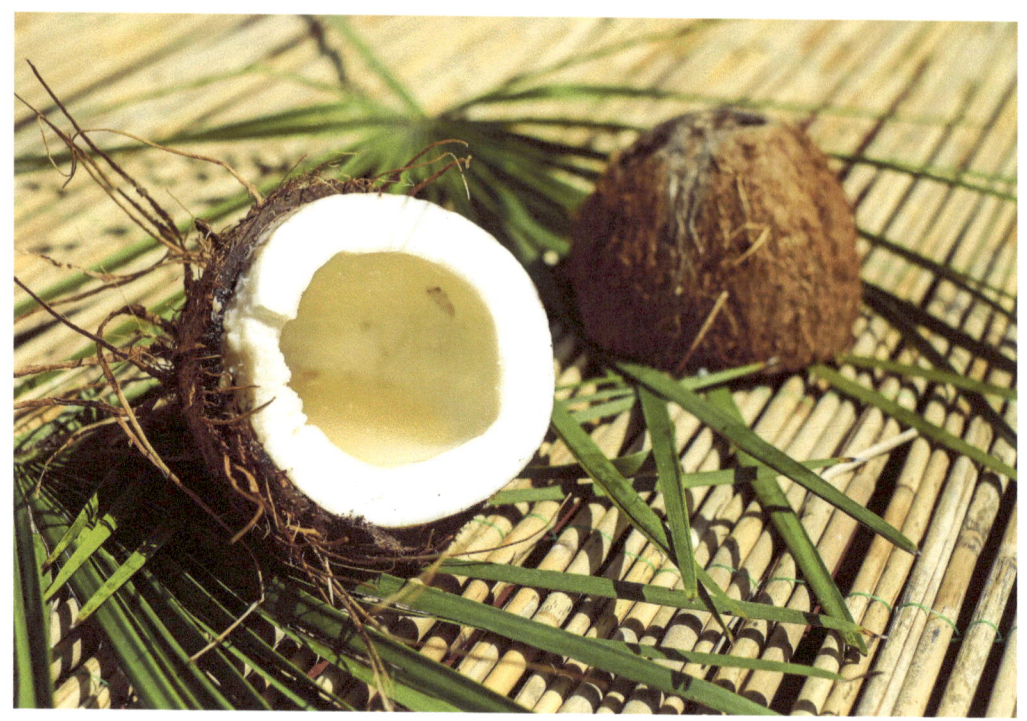

Coconut Mango Butter Lipstick

You will need:

$\frac{1}{2}$ tbs coconut oil
$\frac{1}{3}$ tbs mango butter
$\frac{1}{4}$ tbs Shea butter
$\frac{1}{2}$ tbs beeswax
Powder for color (See list of powders below)

Melt the coconut oil, mango, beeswax and Shea butter in a double boiler. Once melted, add your powder. Put the mixture in a jar or an empty lip gloss container and let it cool in the fridge until it hardens.

List of powders:
Cocoa powder

Paprika powder
Nutmeg powder
Beet powder
Rose powder
Ginger powder
Cinnamon powder
Cumin powder
Natural Mica powder
Eyeshadow
Blush

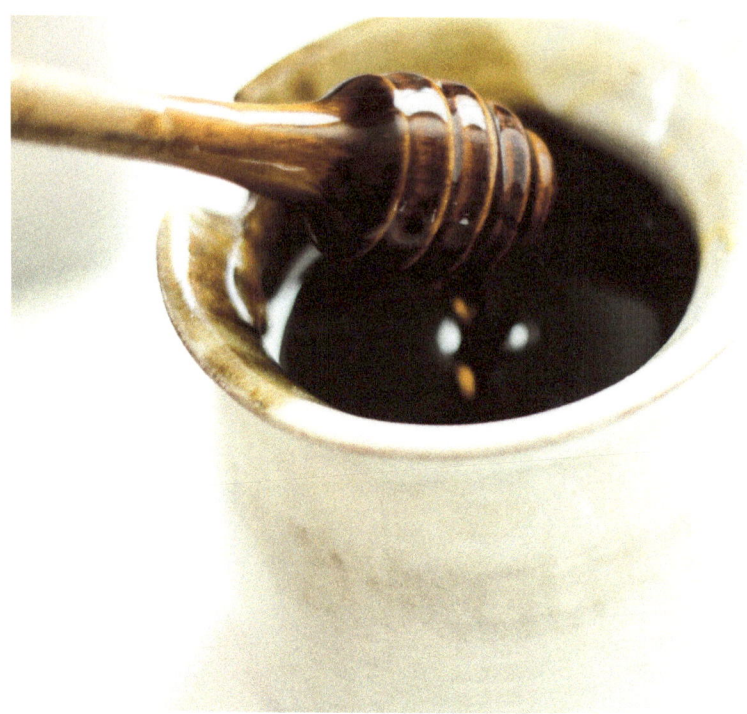

Natural Honey Lipstick

Ensures a light and airy feel without the greasy sensation that Vaseline or heavy beeswax might have.

Start with:

> 1 tbs raw honey
>
> Powder of choice (eyeshadow, blush, natural spices/powders)
>
> ½ tsp olive oil
>
> 1 tbs cocoa butter

Add all of these ingredients to a double boiler and allow them to melt. Once liquified, pour into an empty lip gloss container. Add the powder at this point (play it by eye, the more you add, the more pigmented it will be). Place it in the fridge and let it cool. Must be kept in the fridge at all times or it will melt.

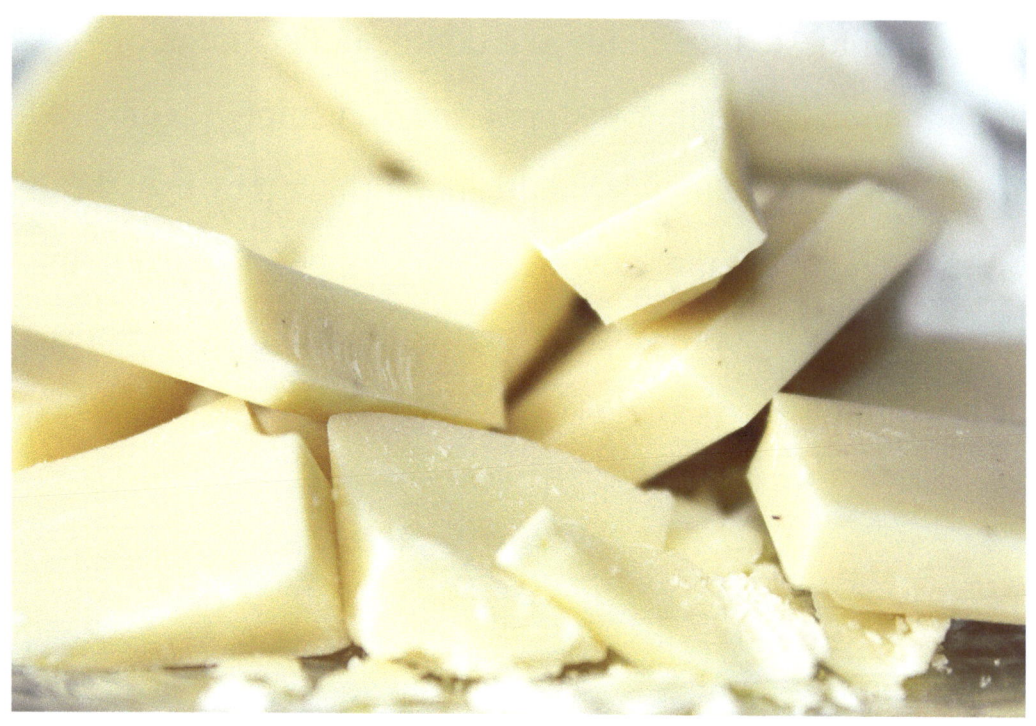

Murumuru Butter Lipstick (restores skin elasticity)

You will need:

½ tbs coconut oil

⅓ tbs murumuru butter

¼ tbs Shea butter

½ tbs beeswax

Melt the ingredients in a double boiler and into an empty lip gloss container. Allow it to cool and harden before applying it to your lips. For color, slowly add powders such as blush, eyeshadow, mica powder, beet powder etc. And as much

as you desire.

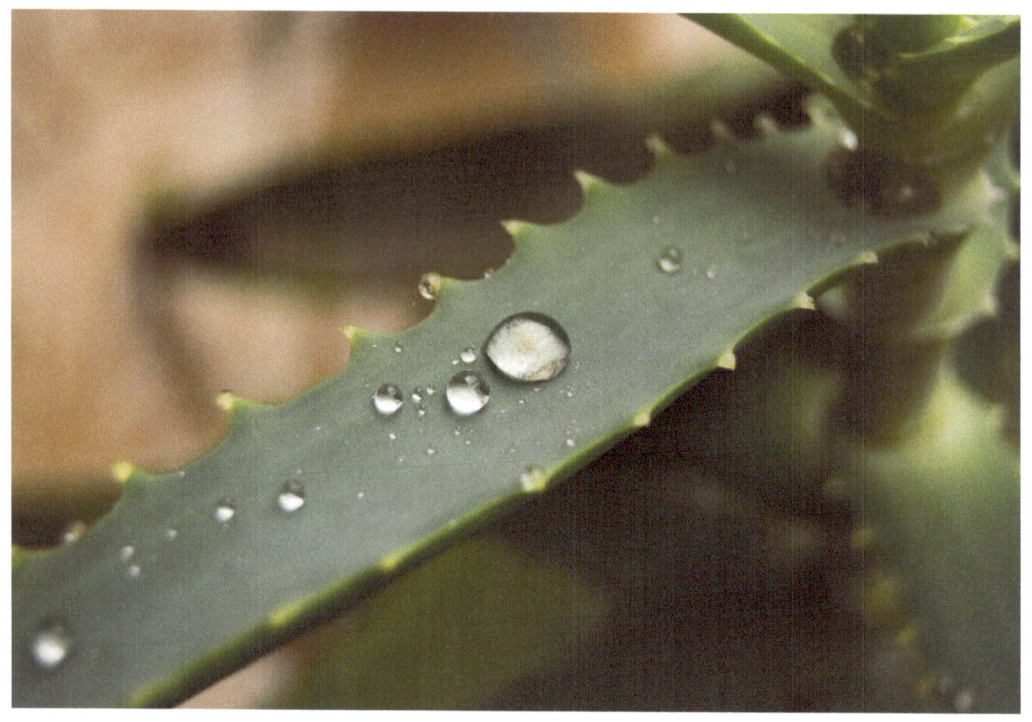

Cocoa Butter And Aloe Lip Gloss

You'll need:

    1 tsp cocoa butter
    1 tsp aloe vera gel from aloe plant
    1 tsp grated beeswax

Melt the cocoa butter and beeswax in a double boiler or

microwave. Once melted, remove from the heat and add in

the aloe vera. Add to a small empty lip gloss container.

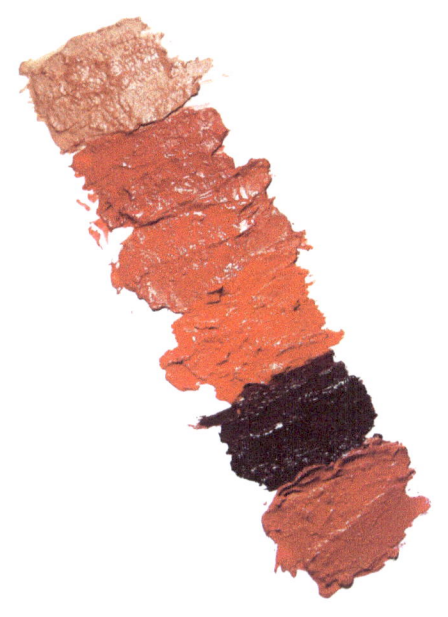

DIY Matte Liquid Lip Gloss

You will need:

    2 pumps or drops of any liquid matte foundation

    1 tsp coconut oil

    Eyeshadow powder of your choice

Mix the foundation and the coconut oil together in an empty lip gloss container. Slowly add your eyeshadow powder until you receive the perfect pigment. The more eyeshadow, the more pigment you will have.

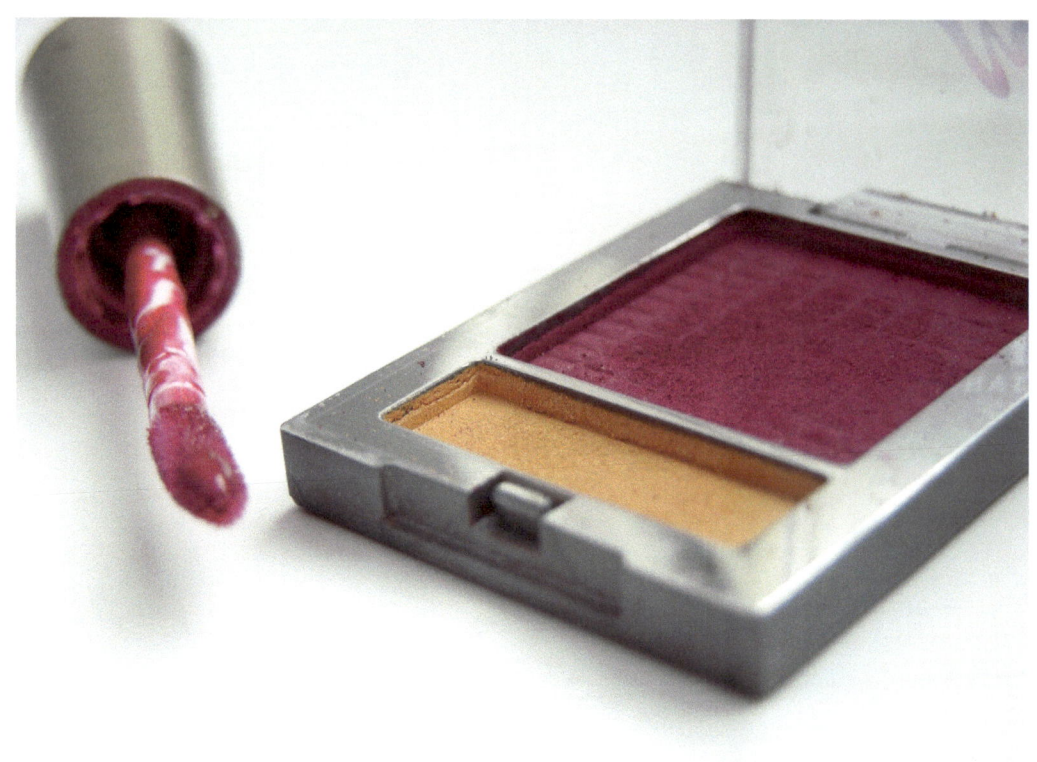

Homemade Dreamy Creamy Lip Gloss

You will need:

Beeswax lip balm

Clear liquid lip gloss

Desired eyeshadow or blush color

Start by scraping off some lip balm and placing it into an empty lip gloss container. Whatever amount of lip balm you added, add twice as much lip gloss. Apply as much eyeshadow or blush powder needed. (The more color you

add, the better). Mix until you are satisfied.

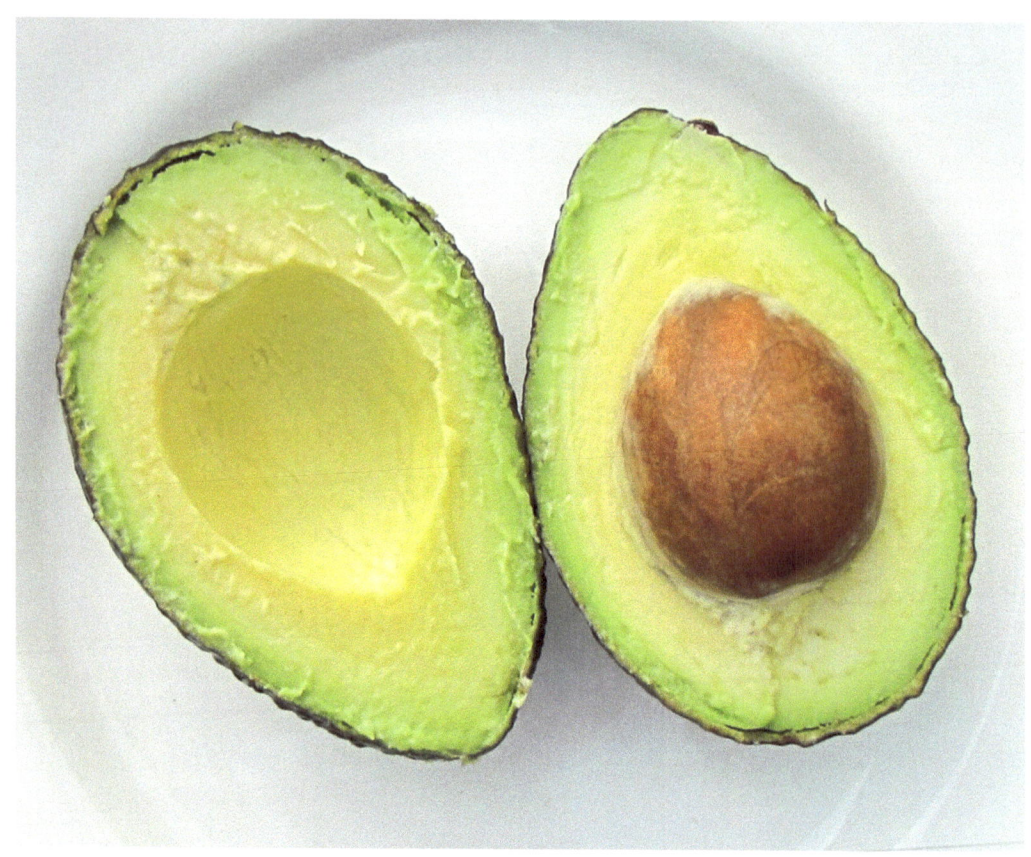

Rich Avocado Lip Gloss

You will need:

½ tbs coconut oil

⅓ tbs avocado butter

¼ tbs Shea butter

½ tbs beeswax

Powder of choice (mica powder, eyeshadow, blush etc.)

Melt the coconut oil, avocado butter, beeswax and shea butter in a double boiler and add your powder once everything has melted. Put it in a jar or an empty lip gloss container and let it cool in the fridge until it hardens.

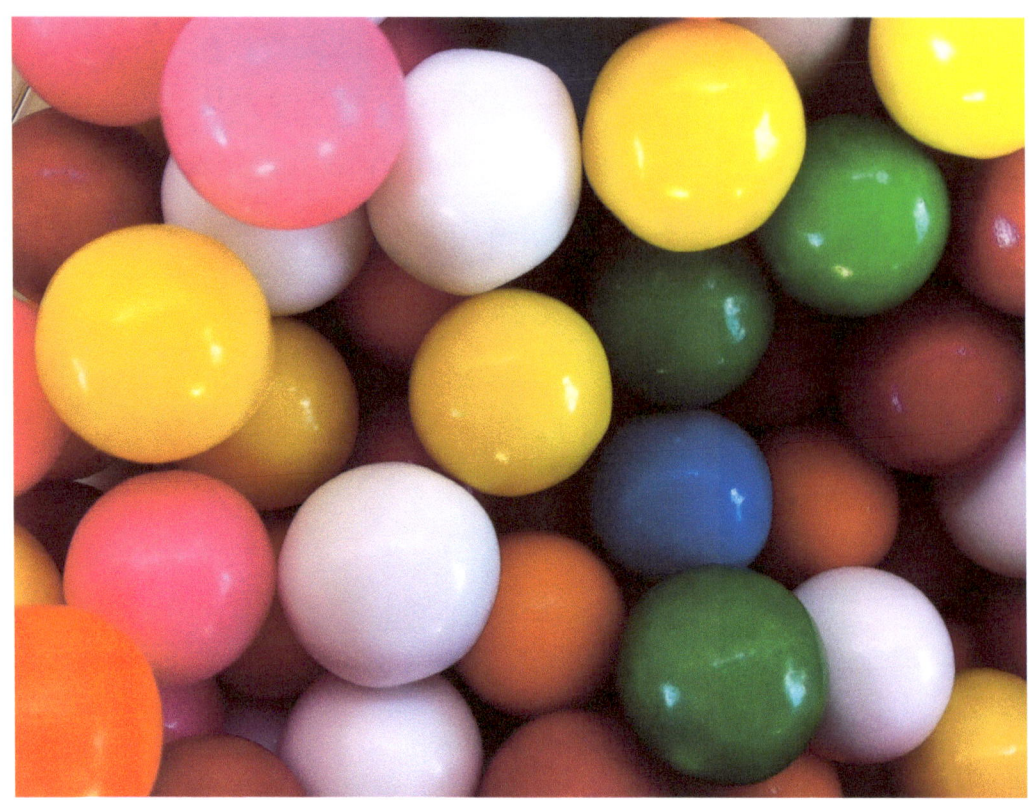

DIY Fun Bubble Gum Lipstick

You will need;

      Two pieces of bubblegum

      1 teaspoon Vaseline

      Food coloring of your choice

Add everything in a bowl and microwave for 30 seconds. Remove and microwave for another 30 seconds. Add to an empty lip gloss container after stirring. Put in the freezer for about 4 to 6 minutes.

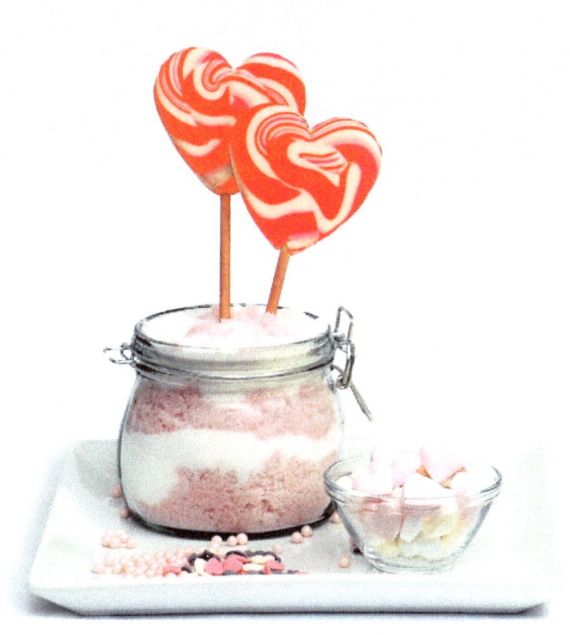

Yummy Sugar Lipstick

In a double boiler, add half a teaspoon of coconut oil, three pieces of beeswax pellets, 1 teaspoon of confectioners sugar and eyeshadow or powder of your choice. Mix everything together once melted and add to an empty lip glass container.

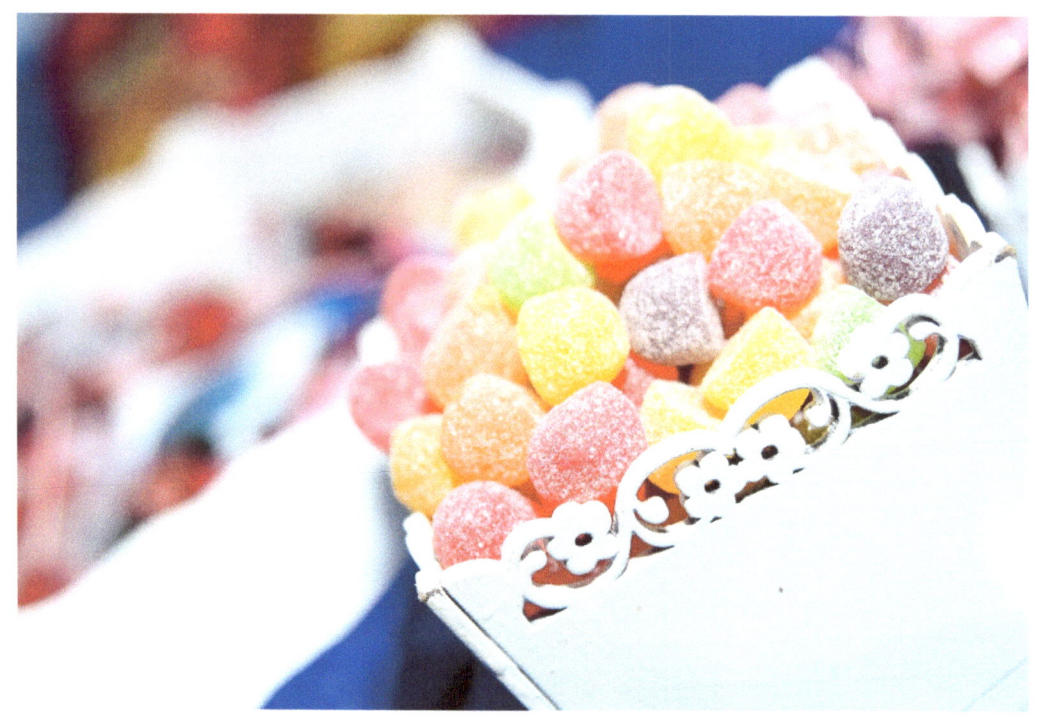

DIY Gummy Candy Lipstick

You will need:

 One gummy candy such as worms, gummy bears, berries etc.

 Half teaspoon coconut oil

 One face painting crayon (the color you desire)

 Glitter eyeshadow

Add all of these ingredients to a double boiler. Only add the glitter once everything has melted and add to an empty lip gloss container.

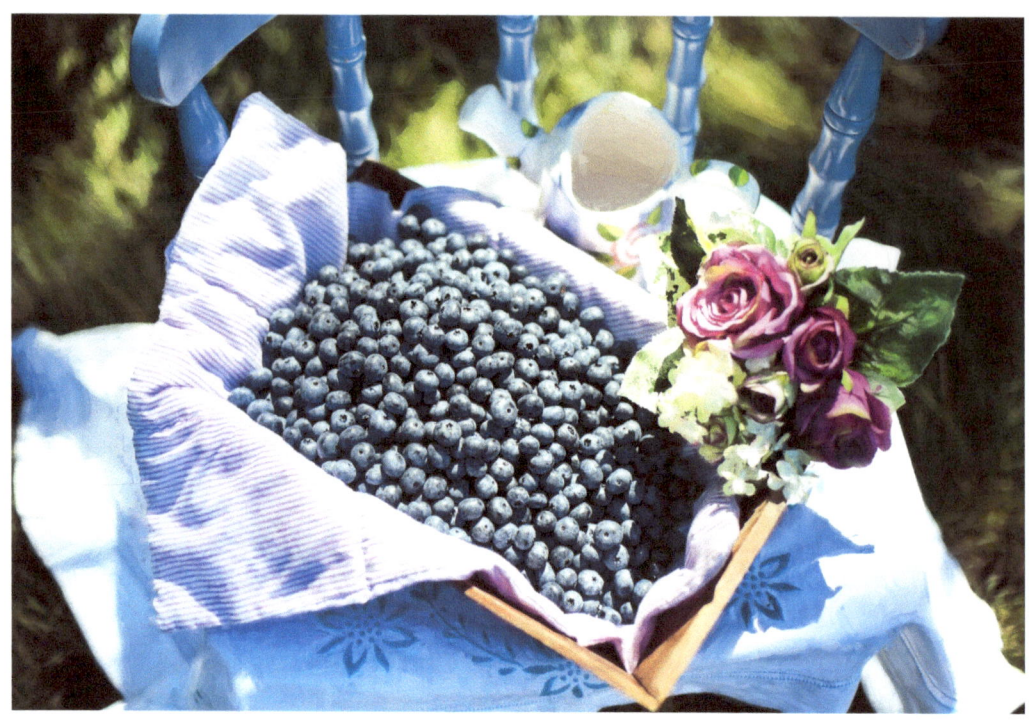

Lipstick Made From Real Fruits And Vegetables

Simply microwave the blueberries and beats for 20 seconds and crush the fruits and vegetables with a fork, in order to liquefy them. Grab a bowl and strain the fruits and vegetables into it. Add 1 teaspoon of Vaseline and microwave in intervals, until ready to add to an empty lip gloss container.

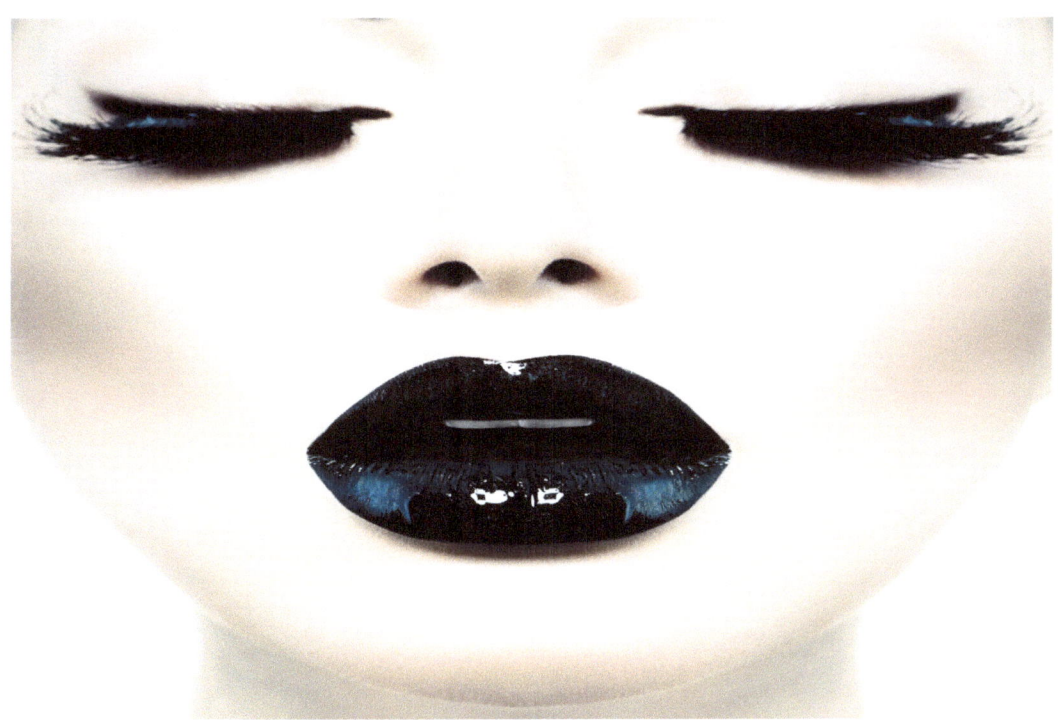

Black Daredevil Lipstick

You will need 1 teaspoon of beeswax cut into tiny pieces, 1 teaspoon of cocoa butter and 1 teaspoon of coconut oil. Add the ingredients into a microwavable bowl and microwave for 30 seconds until melted. Once melted, add 2 capsules of activated charcoal. The more you add, the darker it will be.

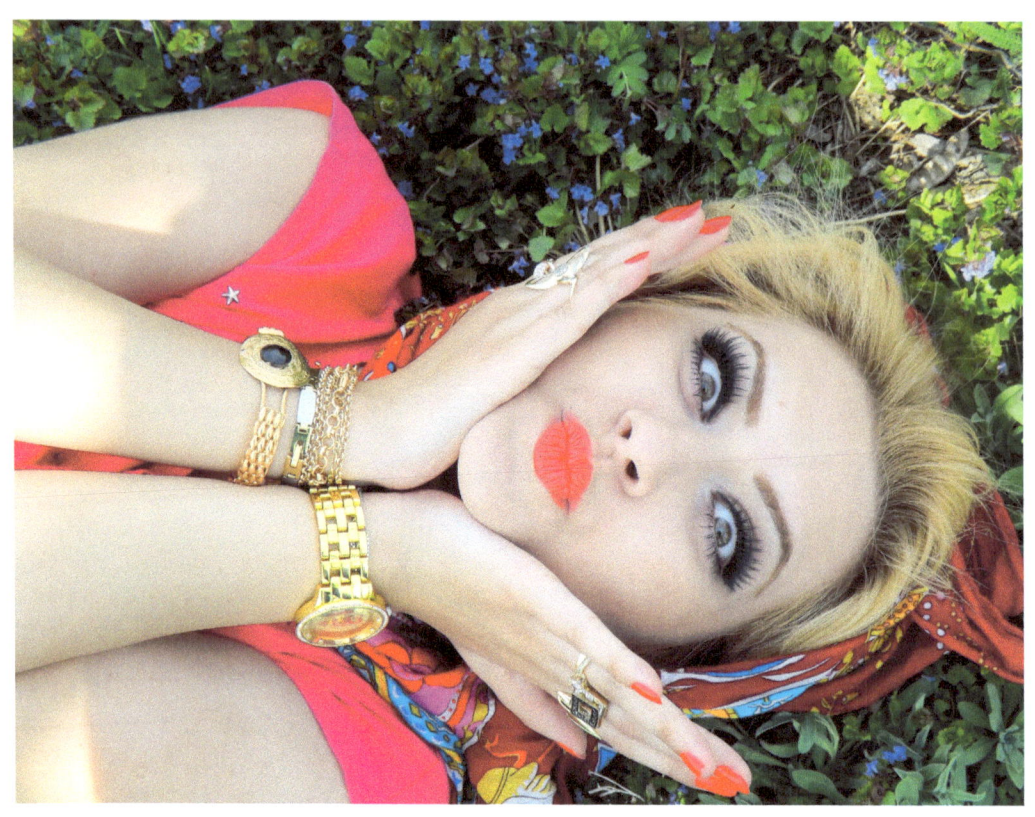

Natural Peppermint Lip Plumper

Add about 1 teaspoon of Vaseline into a bowl, as well as either blush, eyeshadow or mica powder of your choice. Mix the two ingredients together. Add more color for more pigment. Add 2 drops of peppermint extract. Peppermint will cause slight swelling and is known to plump up the lips. It will give the effect of bigger juicier lips.

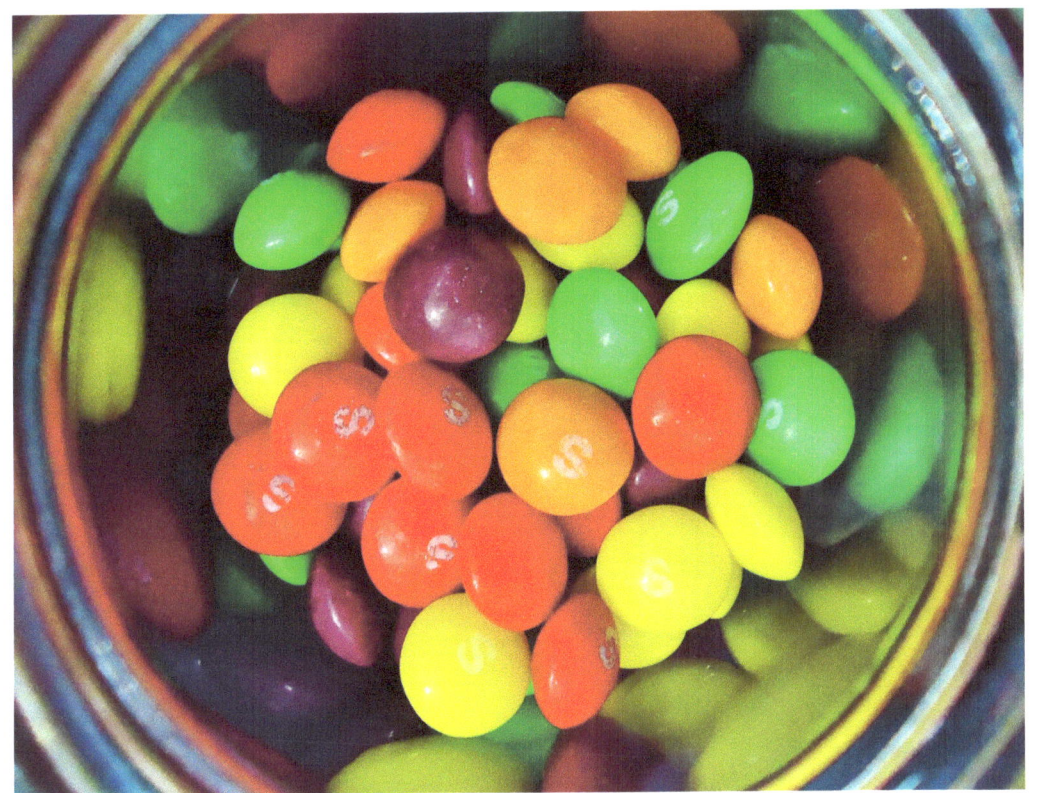

DIY EOS Skittles Lip Balm

You will need:

A cleaned out empty eos lip balm container

10 skittles

A heat safe bowl

Vaseline

Plastic knife

Double boiler

2 tbs water

Disassemble the EOS container. Add the skittles, water and Vaseline to a bowl. Add the bowl into a pot filled with water (double boiler). Once melted, strain any sugar that floats to top of the mixture. Stir and pour into the top of the eos container (not the bottom) and place the eos divider back in. Pour a little more liquid inside, once the divider is placed back in. Place it in the freezer for 3 hours!

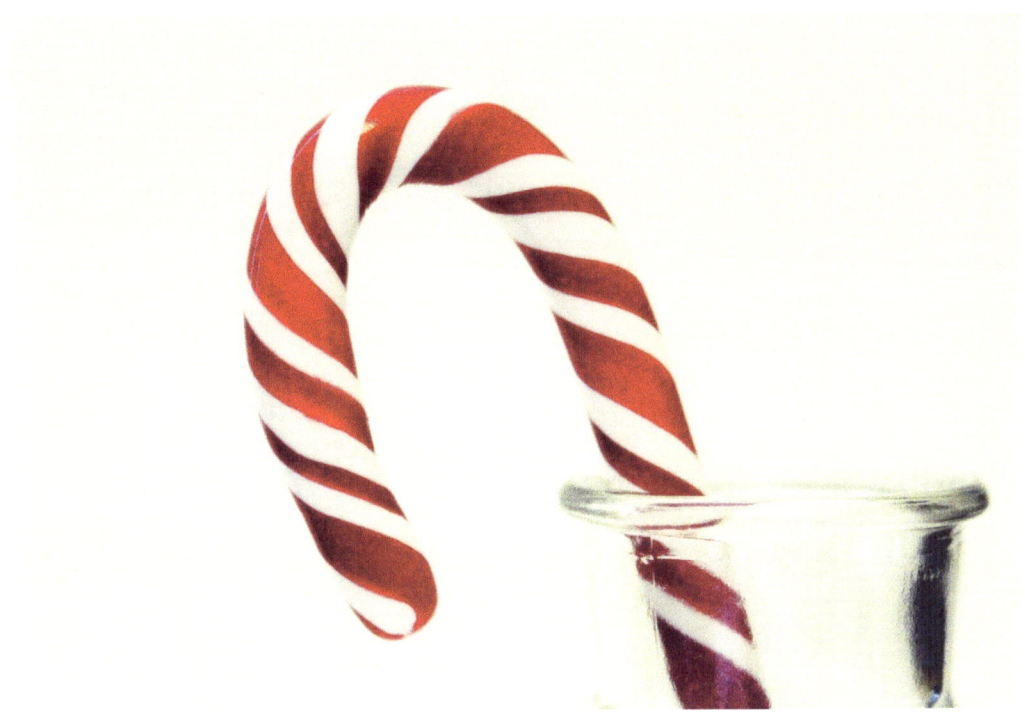

Holiday Special Candy Cane Lip Gloss

You will need:

2 mini heat safe bowls

1 tsp confectioners sugar (x2)

1/2 tsp coconut oil (x2)

1 tsp white eyeshadow or natural powder such as arrowroot

1 tsp red eyeshadow or beet powder

Peppermint extract

Directions:

Place the two heat safe bowls in a double boiler. Add 1/2 tsp of coconut oil in each bowl. Add 3 pellets of beeswax in each bowl. Add the 1 tsp of confectioners sugar in each bowl. Then add 1 tsp white powder in one and 1 tsp of the red in the other. Stir and allow it to melt. Once melted, add the peppermint extract (1-2 drops in each container). Pour the white and red liquid into an empty lip gloss container, alternating both colors, in order to create a candy swirl like effect.

We hope you enjoyed this book and benefited from these unique DIY recipes. Please leave us an Amazon review and let us know what you think! Good Luck!